Functional Strength

Use Resistance Training to Build Strength You Can Actually Use

I0417444

RON KNESS

Contents

Use Resistance Training To Build Strength You Can Actually Use

Chapter 1 – What Is Functional Strength?

Health and fitness fads come and go all the time but unfortunately not all of them are worth your time and effort. Some of them don't work, some of them are overhyped and some of them are just plain dangerous.

But 'functional strength' is different. While functional strength is very much in vogue right now, it's not a 'fad' by any means. In fact, functional strength is the *opposite* of a fad and it's a step in the right direction for all of fitness.

That's because functional strength take it all back: takes it all back to the reasons that most of us started training in the first place. Or at least the reasons we *should* be training.

Because let's be honest: far too many people train 'for the mirror'. How many guys do you see pulling their t-shirt up in front of the mirror after a set of sit-ups? How many women do you see on treadmills wearing the tiniest pants in the world and barely working up a sweat?

Do you think these people are training for the right reasons?

And how about the guy who is so ridiculously muscular that he can't touch his toes any more without busting a gut?

This isn't fitness – not really. And that's what functional strength addresses.

As the name suggests, functional strength is strength that is *functional*. In other words, it's strength that you can *use*. So you're not trying to *look* strong or *look* health – you're trying to *be* those things.

This is the difference between training like a gym bro and training like Bruce Lee. Which would you prefer?

And don't worry if you're not super fit, or if you don't have any interest in becoming an elite athlete: functional strength is important for everyone. Functional strength helps you in every aspect of your life because it gives you better control over your body and your environment. Functional fitness extends to things like flexibility, correct breathing technique and posture. All these things enable you to move with less pain, more grace and more speed.

When you train for functional strength and fitness, *everything* becomes easier: from opening a jam jar, to helping a friend move furniture, to getting out of bed in the morning.

And if you *want* to train for your appearance as your first priority? Well then this is *still* the right way to go: because when you train for strength and power, you look *much* better. Don't believe me? Then think about it logically: the reason that humans find healthy people attractive is because we assume they have better genetics and are better able to protect themselves and their families. Someone with functional strength really *can* do all those things and really *is* healthier – so they send all of those unconscious signals that make them more attractive to the opposite sex!

Why There Are Different Types of Strength

This all sounds great but perhaps you're confused now as to how you can have more than one 'type' of strength. Surely strength is strength... right?

Well to an extent you're right but in other ways... you're not.

To start with, let's take a quick look at 'isolation' training versus 'compound'. Isolation training means that you're specifically training certain muscle groups in isolation – on their own. This is how many of us have been told to train. For instance, when you perform bicep curls, you'll probably do this by holding a dumbbell in one hand and then curling the weight up to meet your shoulder.

This is an isolation movement because the *only* muscle working is the bicep – especially if you're sitting down. Only one joint (the elbow) is moving and everything else is static, thus, one muscle.

But in real life we don't move like this. In real life, nearly every movement from carrying shopping to jumping up steps, requires a combination of muscles working in unison. When you train a bicep curl, you risk building your biceps up *bigger* than the other muscles around them like the triceps and forearms – which can create an imbalance. If your biceps get much bigger than the triceps for instance (which are the antagonistic muscles to the biceps – meaning they apply the opposite force) then this can make the arms look odd and potentially lead to injury. The same goes for leg extensions, hamstring curls, tricep extensions... the list goes on.

Another issue here is that you aren't *teaching* the muscles to work together. Instead, you're using muscles on their own, which means you're more likely to move more efficiently, powerfully and without injury.

A compound movement on the other hand is something like a pull up or a squat. These movements mimic the way we move in real life when climbing or when jumping and that means that they will utilize multiple muscle groups at once in a more efficient and synergistic manner.

When performing any movement in the gym, you should always ask yourself: "when would I use a similar movement in real life?". If you can't think of an answer, then it may mean that the movement you're training isn't actually all that useful and it certainly probably isn't functional!

Training for Strength Vs Size

But that's not the only distinction between training methods either! Another issue to contend with is the difference between training for strength and training for size – because the two are completely different.

If you want to train for strength, then you need to lift heavy weights that are close to your maximum 'one rep max'. This means you're really pushing your body to exert as much power as possible and the more you do this, the more you'll be able to improve your 'mind-muscle' connection, create tears in your muscle fibers (to strengthen them) and improve your technique for generating maximum power.

Use Resistance Training To Build Strength You Can Actually Use

But training for size is a little different. When you train for size, it's much more important to focus on getting 'pump'. This means you're flooding your muscles with blood and metabolites that stimulate growth. The best way to get pump is to use higher repetitions – in other words to use a lighter weight (that you can lift maybe 8-12 times) and to do lots of sets.

The technical terms for these two types of strength training are 'myofibrillar hypertrophy' (strength) and 'sarcoplasmic hypertrophy' (size).

Both *do* have purpose. Training for size also means training for endurance and if you work to build swollen muscles, it means you'll have plenty of fluids in your arms to power you through long workout session. In the real world, this might be the equivalent of carrying heavy bags a long way without fatiguing, so it's certainly useful.

But if you're training like a lot of 'gym bros' you'll only be doing sarcoplasmic training. That means you'll build big muscles sure but it means they won't be as strong as they *could* be.

What You'll Learn in This Book

If you're now starting to feel worried that the training you've been using in the past isn't 'functional', don't worry! That's exactly what we're going to set out to fix in this book, so buckle in and get ready to start training in ways you never imagined. The result? A body that doesn't just look good, but performance like a super-expensive muscle car.

You'll be like a coiled spring, ready to explode into action at any time. Say goodbye to tiredness, to soreness, to weakness – say hello to *functional strength*.

Specifically we'll be looking at:

- Functional training methods
- Tools and techniques
- Stretching
- Injury prevention
- Diet strategies
- MovNat
- Bodyweight training
- And much more!

Chapter 2 – The 7 Primal Movements

The unfortunate fact of the matter is that most of us, gym bro or not, are not 'functional'. The vast majority of us find it difficult to move around in our environment, suffer from bad backs and knee pain and aren't all that strong.

This is a result of the way we live. Unfortunately, modern life is not conducive to functional fitness because we're very rarely challenged physically in any meaningful way. The majority of us spend most of our time sitting down and that means we're getting zero exercise.

What makes this worse though, is that sitting itself is actually bad for us too.

Why? Because when we sit, we're forced into an unnatural position. Think about it: there were no chairs in the wild and you never would have made this movement.

When you sit at a desk, it forces your legs into a right angle. This then means that your hip flexors – the muscles that move your legs upward in front of you – will be shortened and tightened. At the same time, your hip extensors found around the back, will be stretched and elongated.

Meanwhile, your pecs are also going to be bunched up as your arms lean forward and your neck will be constantly pointing down at the screen. Your back will likely be rounded too, shoulders forward and diaphragm squashed by the weight of your upper body.

In other words: you're gradually destroying your joints and musculature. *And you sit like this for 8 hours a day, 5 days a week!*

Then you come home and sit like it some more!

So how would we relax in the wild? Simple: we'd squat. Squatting is the natural equivalent of sitting and it's actually really good for us because it puts us in a full body stretch. Today, a fair proportion of people are actually *incapable* of squatting at all. Try it yourself: are you able to completely squat down while keeping your heel flat on the floor?

This is considered one of the basic, fundamental movements that *all* of us should be able to do. In fact, there are thought to be seven of these 'primal movements' which are:

- Squatting
- Lunging
- Bending
- Pushing
- Pulling
- Gait (walking or running)
- Twisting

If you can't do these basic seven things, then chances are that you're lacking in fitness, in flexibility and in general health – and it will very likely lead to injury and other problems somewhere down the line.

So can you guess where we're going to go with this? That's right: these are the basic movements that a good training program should be made up of. By training the 7 primal movements, you're able to strengthen yourself through all the regular movements that you might face in daily life and you're able to prevent injury in all of them.

And now, if you introduce additional isolation exercise on top of this just to 'hone' a particular muscle group that seems to be lagging, then you'll be able to improve your aesthetics without worrying about creating imbalances or potentially encouraging an injury.

Compound Movements and Big Lifts

We briefly touched on the idea of compound movements in the introduction but just to reiterate: these are your movements that utilize multiple major muscle groups at once in unison. Examples of compound lifts include:

- Squat
- Deadlift
- Bench press
- Pull up
- Press up
- Overhead press
- Kettlebell swing

What's also cool about these movements, is that they actually lead to better fat loss and muscle gain. That's because the body responds to us training our muscles by producing a variety of hormones called 'anabolic hormones'. These include growth hormone and testosterone, which in turn tell the body to start burning fat and building muscle tissue.

The more muscle you use, the more of these hormones get released. So as you can imagine, something like the squat that incorporates all of your biggest muscles into one powerful movement, will *really* encourage your body to go into a muscle-building zone.

What's also key to point out at this stage, is that compound movements also allow you to lift heavier weights. Why? Because when you go compound, you're using *more big muscle*. More big muscle means more power, means more weight! And as you might imagine, the more weight you move, the more intense the workout becomes for the body as a whole.

Compound Lifts Are for Everyone!

If you're a guy and you want to build massive muscles that looked ripped and shredded beneath a very low body fat percentage, then compound lifts are the *number one* strategy you should be using.

But that's not the only demographic that these movements are ideal for. Just as importantly, women should also be using compound lifts. Just Google 'girls who squat' and you'll see some of the most impressively formed buttocks on the web.

Use Resistance Training To Build Strength You Can Actually Use

As mentioned, those all-important anabolic hormones that get released when you lift heavy weights don't *only* result in building more muscle. Likewise, they also help you to burn more fat to get a leaner look.

In fact, lifting weights – and especially using compound movements – is one of the very best ways to burn fat and to lower your bodyfat percentage overall. That's because it doesn't *only* burn calories *while* you're training, but also encourages your body to continue burning calories throughout the days and weeks that follow. Simply *having* muscle requires the body to burn fat simply to sustain that mass.

If you're a woman trying to get into shape and you've spent years running for miles and eating barely anything, then your hormones probably aren't working in your favor. Get down to the gym, start lifting, and you might well see results start coming faster.

And finally we have those who are suffering with joint pains and mobility issues. Perhaps you're elderly, perhaps you're recovering from some kind of injury. Both way, you find it difficult to get around and you're thinking that maybe you shouldn't be lifting heavy weights...

Well, you probably don't need to be lifting *really* heavy weights but there's nothing wrong with taking some lighter ones and still training these compound movements. Using compound lifts like these train your body to move correctly and this is an excellent way to restore mobility and health.

Some Moves to Get You Started

So with that in mind, what are some compound movements that you can use to start targeting the seven primal movements? Here are some examples.

- Squatting – Squats, deadlifts, kettlebell swings
- Lunging – Lunges, side squats
- Bending – Deadlifts, sit ups, leg raises
- Pushing – Bench press, overhead press, push up
- Pulling – Pull up, row
- Gait– Jogging, running, walking
- Twisting – Heavy bag, twisting sit ups, cable woodchop

So, if you take these exercises and combine them into a workout, you'll have performed a routine that targeted every important movement the human body is capable of, that recruits a huge amount of muscle and that puts the body into a highly anabolic state.

Important: Before you try any of these movements, it's important that you learn to do them properly. This is kind of *the whole point*. If you don't learn how to use the moves properly then you'll actually just be rehearsing and learning bad movement patterns, which will in turn cause you to become increasingly injury prone. Little mistakes like rounding the back during a squat can even lead to an immediate injury so make sure you find a trainer in the gym or someone who looks like they know what they're doing and ask for help.

You can find plenty of instruction online but nothing beats actually speaking with someone who can see your form and correct it in person.

Chapter 3 – Relax Into Stretch And Foam Rolling

Something you might notice when trying these movements though is that… you can't. Or at least you can't very confidently.

This will be a result of all those years of sitting at your desk and not doing anything. So how do you get back some basic mobility and learn to move properly again? One thing that can help a great deal is to practice stretching, in which case you'll be able to regain your full range of motion.

So how do you go about doing that?

How to 'Relax Into Stretch'

According to Pavel Tsatsouline, the vast majority of us go about this the wrong way entirely. If you're used to stretching by forcing yourself into a position until it hurts, then you may actually be doing more harm than good. So stop it right away!

How do we know this is a bad move? Well, it can be demonstrated with a simple bit of self-experimentation. Simply lie on the ground on one side of your body so one arm and one leg are touching the floor beneath you.

Now, raise your leg up 90 degrees to point right at the ceiling. It should be fairly easy.

Now roll onto the other side and raise the opposite leg up again. Easy, yes?

So if you can move both legs to 90 degrees, why can't you do the box splits?

It's got nothing to do with any 'tissue' connecting your legs either. In fact, there is no tissue other than bone between your legs – no ligaments and no muscle to prevent you from doing the splits.

According to Pavel then, what's actually happening is that your brain is forcing you to stop before you reach box splits in order to try and prevent an injury. Again, it comes down to the fact that you don't normally utilize this amount of flexibility, which teaches your brain and body that it's bad news.

More specifically, it comes down to your central nervous system, which is responsible for all the 'knee jerk reactions' of your musculature that lie outside the domain of your conscious control. It's also your CNS that is responsible for your eye blinking when someone is trying to get an eyelash out of it.

Years of training yourself to believe that you *can't* do box splits and years of moving within a far more limited range of movement have taught your body to 'lock' in place when you try and move outward.

So guess what happens if you try and force yourself into a split? That's right: your body fights back by tensing up your muscles and making it even more difficult. And you further teach your body that it can't go into that position.

Instead then, the better technique is to much more gently ease yourself into these positions and then to actively relax your body as much as possible. Move to the point where it just starts to hurt and then relax your body as much as possible. The more you do this, the more you'll remove that knee-jerk reaction and you'll regain your *natural* flexibility.

Note that you *shouldn't* use this kind of training for your back – so don't use it when touching your toes. We're actually *meant* to be limited in some of our movements and if you override this it can lead to injury.

But for movements involving the legs and the arms, this technique can be *highly* useful and many people find that it helps them to regain their movement in no time at all.

More Fixes for Mobility and Flexibility

For the back meanwhile, yoga can be an incredible tool for improving your ability to move. In fact, yoga is something that pretty much everyone should do and if you combine it with the techniques recommended by Pavel and a training program full of compound lifts, you'll be on your way to increased mobility in no time.

And don't get this twisted. If you're thinking now that stretching isn't going to make much difference to you, or that it's somehow 'for girls' then you've got another thing coming. If you feel tired and lethargic, or if you feel stiff, then you *need* stretching. Stretching will not only help you to remove pain and discomfort; it will help you to feel far more full of child-like energy than you have done for years. You'll find you're faster and more mobile and more ninja-like in general.

Stretching all makes us stronger. Studies show that people who stretch regularly are able to lift heavier weights, which in turn is likely because the muscles and ligaments themselves present less resistance when they try to lift. They're not fighting their own body as well as the weights.

But note that you actually shouldn't stretch just prior to a workout. Contrary to popular belief, this actually makes you weaker *and* more prone to injury by removing some of the tension that keeps your muscles in place and where they should be. Stretch *after* workouts or as part of a separate program performed on its own.

Meanwhile, you should also look into self-myofascial release. This is another health 'fad' that's found its way into the gym that's nevertheless something you should pay attention to. Self-myofascial release is what you might also know as foam rolling (though it can also use a tennis ball). This basically involves rolling around on something solid that will protrude into the fascia and help to remove knots and 'fascial adhesions'.

How to Use Foam Rolling

Without getting into too much science here, the fascia is essentially a large piece of tissue that looks like a thin 'film' and that surrounds all of your muscles and joints. It's a bit like your muscles have all been vacuum packed and this is what keeps everything in place while at the same time supporting you through movements to avoid movement.

Use Resistance Training To Build Strength You Can Actually Use

The fascia is something that modern science is only just getting around to looking at but it's thought by many to be as important, if not *more* important that the musculature itself.

When you contract your muscle, your brain sends impulses through your nervous system. Once these impulses reach your motor end plates, they release calcium among other things to tell the fibers to begin contracting. The body needs to remove this calcium over time but sometimes this doesn't go as smoothly as it should and the resultant build up leaves the muscles contracting in single points. This creates a tiny localized bulge of tension that can inhibit movement and create pain.

Fascial adhesions meanwhile are caused when the fascia is torn or damaged and ends up forming a more rigid, less flexible scar tissue. The fascia doesn't show up on MRI scans, so often this damage goes completely unrecognized – but it causes painful movement and other problems and needs to be dealt with.

Foam rolling is essentially like giving yourself a sports massage that really gets right into those fascial adhesions and knots in order to work them out and give you back your movement.

To do it, you need to get yourself a foam roller or a tennis ball and then roll your back and other muscles across it. Move it around directly on the muscle until you feel a sudden twinge of pain. It should hurt but it should feel like 'good pain' that's somewhat satisfying at the same time.

Self-myofascial release *can* be used right before a workout and should also have the same benefits for increasing strength during lifts.

Chapter 4 – Functional Strength Training Tools: Kettlebells, Indian Clubs and More

So far your training regime consists of lots of compound movements, alongside some relaxed stretching and self-myofascial release. Congratulations! Your training program is *already* far superior to that of half the people in the gym and will be better for your functional strength and your overall health and fitness.

But there's just one problem... it's pretty boring!

Notice how in the real world, we don't find ourselves doing the same five things over and over again. In fact, in the real world our 'form' on each movement is completely different every time we do anything. You don't really squat in the wild, but rather you would pick up randomly shaped boulders. Likewise, you'd be forced to do pull ups on branches that were completely the wrong shape and size or you'd have to run across uneven terrain. Then fight a lion... (maybe).

In other words, training should be constantly changing and varied if it's really going to mimic the real world and if it's really going to be 'functional'.

So how do you ensure your workouts fit that bill? Simple: you introduce some interesting tools and techniques that will mix things up for you.

Here are some cool examples...

Kettlebells

Kettlebells have grown to become some of the most popular tools for use in the gym as more and more people have been waking up to the importance of functional strength.

The kettlebell is essentially a weight that can be used like dumbbell but which has an entirely different shape. Specifically, the dumbbell is shaped like an iron ball with a handle poking out of the top. What this means, is that when you lift it, the weight is *below* your arm. That now means that it's capable of swinging and of creating its own momentum, which you then have to control and fight against in order to perform repetitions. This then forces you to use your core in what would otherwise be relatively isolated movements. Likewise, it challenges you to lift at awkward angles and to generate power in unexpected ways.

All in all, kettlebells are more functional than dumbbells and provide some interesting new training options.

But perhaps their most important use is the kettlebell swing. This is a movement that involves clasping the handle with both hands and then swinging the weight between your legs while going through a squatting and 'popping' movement.

This then mimics the movement you use when you perform deadlifts but means you don't need to find space in your house for a whole barbell that you'll be dropping repeatedly on the floor.

It also means that the exercise is much faster, which turns it into a great fat-burning move as well as a muscle-building one.

When you combine these benefits, the kettlebell is alone one of the most versatile and important pieces of training equipment in your arsenal.

Indian Club Training

Off the back of the kettlebell has come another very popular piece of training equipment: the Indian club. The Indian club doesn't look like anything special; rather it looks like a stick with a heavy ball on the end of it. Like the kettlebell though, its strength lies in its awkwardness. When you wave around the Indian club, the weight isn't where your brain expects it to be and you're essentially lifting it against a long lever arm. These combined factors mean that you're once again forced to engage your core and your grip if you want to keep it under control. The Indian club is great fun and an awesome training tool if you have a garden. If you use it in the hoes though, you can expect to smash just about everything you own...

And this brings us to another interesting option: which is to just use the stuff lying around your house. You don't have to spend money on fancy training equipment because almost everything in your house is unevenly weighted and can be turned into a piece of workout equipment. A great example? A chair that's strong enough to be lifted and swung around.

Here once again, the weight is much greater at the end and if you hold the top of it, you'll be forced to engage all kinds of muscles just to keep it in place.

Barefoot Running

Another craze that has taken off alongside the whole functional movement... is that of barefoot running.

Barefoot running means taking off your shoes before going jogging, normally through a rural environment of trails that challenge you to jump over ditches and dodge around roots and stones. When you do this, your toes are able to splay across the ground that prevents you from falling over or twisting your ankle while simultaneously letting you use the small muscles in your foot to propel yourself forward.

Barefoot running should be able to help you improve your gait as well, by forcing you to land with the ball of your foot when you land. This cushions your fall more than hitting the floor with your heel first (as most of us do) and allows the leg to bend like a leopard's, in the foot, in the ankle, in the knee and at the hip.

Of course barefoot running doesn't always mean going *completely* bare footed as that wouldn't be very wise anywhere were you could step on glass or sharp stones. Instead, you can use barefoot shoes like the Vibram Five Fingers. These offer pockets for your toes, allowing them to move freely but also offering just enough protection to keep you safe.

TRX

Another very exciting piece of equipment you can use for training in a functional manner is TRX. TRX is a device that can attach to a pull up bar (which you can get for your doorframe for about $10) and which then gives you suspension straps you can rest your hands and feet on. This then allows you to perform all kinds of cool moves, from bodyweight rows (holding onto the handles and pulling your upper body toward the bar) to suspended push-ups and bodyweight dips (both of which force you to stabilize your body as the handles wobble around).

But don't actually buy TRX. Why? Because TRX costs about $200 and you can get the very same thing with a pair of gymnastic rings. Gymnastic rings that will cost you all of about $20 and which are actually more versatile.

Important: Once again, it's important at this juncture to mention some health and safety. Injury to the shoulder is common with TRX/gymnastic rings. Likewise, injury to the knee is common with barefoot running (and Vibrams).

That's not to say these aren't good for you, it just means that you have to be careful and introduce them slowly into your routine while taking care to get proper instruction.

Chapter 5 – Bodyweight Training for Strength-to-Weight Ratio

TRX and gymnastic rings mix things up a little because they involve bodyweight training instead of lifting weights. Bodyweight training is actually *ideal* for general fitness and for functional strength in particular. The reason is that bodyweight training means you have to lift your *own* body – something that we regularly have to do in real life. If you can get stronger faster than you get heavier, then you can increase your strength-to-weight ratio and that in turn will make you far faster on your feet as well as more agile and flexible.

Another advantage of bodyweight training is that it forces you to utilize all the smaller supportive muscles in your body. When you perform a press-up, you are using muscle in your abs, obliques, legs, lower back and more to keep your body rigid and in position. The same is true when you perform a pull-up – and if you try and cheat through the pull-up, then your body will wobbly around in the air and you'll end up wasting energy and tiring out faster.

This gets far more impressive as you start to approach more advanced movements. Imagine the kind of total-body control that is used when you perform a handstand press-up, or planche press-ups (press-ups where your feet don't touch the ground!).

If you want to see an example of someone who is truly in command of their own body and their own strength, then look up 'Ido Portal'.

He moves like an inhuman and will blow your mind regarding the potential of the human body.

How to Approach Bodyweight Training

The problem is that many people approach bodyweight training all wrong. If you're just pumping out a set number of press-ups and sit-ups every day, then you can't expect to progress much. Instead, you should be challenging yourself with increasingly difficult moves in your 8-10 rep range and you should be using techniques to push past failure.

In bodyweight routines you can't change the weight itself but what you change instead is the way you're lifting it — which can be just as challenging.

Find press-ups easy? Then how about training with clapping press-ups and trying to launch yourself in the air? This move requires acceleration in the muscles, which the body treats just the same as heavy weight. The result is that you'll recruit more of your fast-twitch muscle fibers in order to explode off the floor.

And *now* if you try and perform some 'normal' push-ups, you'll find it's a lot more challenging.

Likewise, if you perform a push-up with one hand, that will also make it harder, as well as requiring you to strengthen your core to avoid tipping. You can build up to this by placing both hands on the floor but putting 80% of your weight on one hand.

As you get more tired, move more and more weight onto the other side. Now you're controlling your distribution of weight in order to maximally challenge the muscle.

You can also just move your arms back closer to your waist, which puts you in a position called a 'maltese push-up'. This movement lengthens the lever arm – just like the Indian club. Now your weight is further away from your hands, which forces you to work harder.

The Mechanical Drop Set and Progressions

A great tool at your disposal here is a technique called the 'mechanical drop set'. Here, you perform as many reps as you can of an exercise and then make it slightly easier by changing the position. For instance, you might do as many pushups as you can and then change immediately to press-ups on your knees. This enables you to go past the point of failure but still keep going, which makes it much harder.

And in terms of each workout, the goal is to keep challenging yourself to perform more and more difficult movements which are called 'progressions'. Once you can easily do 10 maltease push-ups, you can then challenge yourself to do a single planche push-up.

Ultimately, you should aim to get to the point where you're performing feats of 'hand balancing' which will involve moving from one impressive bodyweight position on your hands to another, all in a slow, controlled manner.

Chapter 6 – Overcoming Isometrics and Grip Strength

As you incorporate these techniques into your training, you should find yourself beginning to gain in strength and mobility.

There's another piece of the puzzle that's missing though and if you don't incorporate it, you will be limiting your potential progress. That's 'grip strength', which you need in order to improve every other lift in the gym and all your bodyweight moves.

The true kings of functional strength are the 'old-time strongmen' of old. These guys would lift insane amounts of weight in all kinds of unusual manners – such as lifting barbells over their head with just one hand. The 'anyhow lift' was a lift that challenged a man to life as much weight as he possibly good with any technique he wanted!

And key to the training of these old-time strongmen was grip strength. Why? Because they knew it was the key to being able to move weight around more confidently. And this is something that you need to learn as well.

To train your grip, you need to simply incorporate some grip training into your workouts. You can do this with towel pull ups for instance, or by doing pull ups on a finger board. Likewise, you can also use bars that are slightly wider for your other lifts. You won't be able to lift as much but you'll get a far more impressive full-body workout that will increase your *true* strength.

Overcoming Isometrics

Better yet, you can also try using overcoming isometrics – which are a type of training used by some of the strongest men in the world even today. Bruce Lee used overcoming isometrics and so does Dennis Rogers – pound for pound the strongest man alive (Dennis is so strong that he appeared on *Stan Lee's: Superhumans!*)

So what is overcoming isometrics?

Well, isometric training is any kind of training that involves no movement at all. This is the opposite of dynamic training or of plyometric training (the latter of which involves exploding up out of the movement).

There are two kinds of isometric training. One is 'yielding' which means you simply hold a position that is quite tough but not impossible until you wilt. An example would be plank, where you hold the plank position for about 2-3 minutes.

The other type of isometric training, the one we're looking at now, is 'overcoming'. Here, you're attempting to lift a weight that's too much for you and then just pushing against it as hard as you can. In fact, it doesn't even have to be a weight; you can even just press against a wall and try and push it down!

When you do this, your body recruits as much of your muscle fiber as it can and treats the challenge as though you were trying to lift 100% of your one-rep max. As far as your muscles are concerned they're maxed out and it makes no difference if anything is moving or not.

The result is that the brain tries to recruit *all* of your strength – which doesn't normally happen – and learns that it needs greater control over your muscle fiber. The result is that your mind-muscle connection strengthens and the next time you try this move, you should have developed the ability to move more weight.

You can't train with *just* this type of training because it doesn't involve any 'range of motion'. But as a compliment to compound lifts, it can greatly increase your power. What's more, is that many of the best types of overcoming isometric training do involve the grip.

And example? Trying to bend an iron bar. Don't have an iron bar around? Then how about trying to roll up a frying pan. Or just crush a stress ball?

If you want to use something that feels a little more rewarding, try investing in a power twister. These are bars that have a powerful spring in the middle and let you bend them to train your crushing power. They go all the way up to 100KG so they can provide an amazing challenge!

Chapter 7 - HIIT

Now you know how to train your strength and increase fitness but to be truly 'functional' you need to be fit as well.

This is where HIIT comes in.

HIIT is 'High Intensity Interval Training' and simply put, it is the more effective successor to 'steady state cardio'.

Steady state cardio is running for 40 minutes and then calling it a day. This exhausts your body and your joints but actually it doesn't challenge your cardiovascular system as much as some other kinds of training. Conversely, in HIIT, you train by using intervals of high intensity followed by intervals of relative rest called 'active recovery'.

So instead of running at a steady pace for forty minutes, instead you sprint at nearly 100% exertion for 1 minute, jog for three minutes and then repeat. The first great thing about HIIT training is that it's much quicker: in about 15 minutes you can get the equivalent workout to 40 minutes or running or more. This is great if you're someone who isn't a particularly big fan of running for long periods because it means you can burn a ton of fat in a much shorter amount of time and in a manner that's easier to stick to.

Moreover though, is that HIIT is both more effective at burning fat *and* more useful for general life and thereby more functional.

When you use HIIT, what happens is that during the intense exertion stage, your body is forced to use up all the immediately available glucose in your blood. This is because you're in an 'anaerobic state' meaning that you're working out too hard for your body to burn fat for fuel in time.

This might sound like a bad thing but in the long run it's good because it means that come the next round of exercise – the active recovery – your body now has *only* fat stores to burn for fuel. This then makes it considerably more efficient at burning fat for the remainder of the workout and at the same time, forces your body to continue burning fat throughout the day subsequently. Like training compound movements it's not only about the amount of calories you're burning in the short term, but also the amount of calories that you continue to burn as a result of that kind of training.

There's another benefit to HIIT from a functional standpoint too, which is that it challenges you to burn fat for energy as quickly as possible. As with anything in training, the best way to get better at something is to challenge your body to do it under tougher circumstances. As a result, this is a great tool for increasing your body's efficiency and energy metabolism. In particular, HIIT increases the efficiency and the number of mitochondria in your cells. These are the 'energy factories' that the body uses to convert glucose into ATP (useable energy) and as such, getting more of them is one of the most effective ways to burn more fat and to feel more energetic.

In fact, studies suggest that the difference in mitochondria may be the main reason that young children have so much more energy than elderly people. No form of training is capable of increasing mitochondria count and function to the same extent as HIIT and this makes it an incredibly valuable tool for anyone who wants to improve their performance and their general health.

Chapter 8 – Is There Any Place Left For Resistance Machines?

As you can see, there is a new guard coming in when it comes to fitness and the whole approach is different than it ever has been. More research and better education have taught us that you can't approach weight training simply by pumping iron until your muscles get bigger: you need to think about how it affects your physiology and your movement.

So with all that in mind, the question is: is there any place left for traditional weightlifting? More specifically, is there any place left for resistance machines?

Resistance Machines, What Are They Good For?

In case you're in the dark at this point, a resistance machine is essentially any piece of equipment that guides you through a workout. They're often take up a large proportion of the gym and have more space dedicated to them than the 'free weights' (tragically). Usually they're white and in most cases they utilize some kind of pulley system in order to move weights around.

You sit yourself down on a comfortable seat, you push a metal pin into a rack of weights to set how much you want to use... and then you get lifting! By pushing the handle, pulling the cable or moving some kind of appendage, a hinge guides you through a very specific range of motion and this then ensures that you train the target muscle.

Now, if you've been paying attention, you should *already* be able to see what's wrong with this approach. This is the *opposite* of compound and the opposite of functional. This is even *more* isolated than a seated dumbbell curl! Your arm is being guided through a specific arc of movement and there is *literally* no way you can deviate from this path. No other muscles are being used other than to brace you in the chair and you don't even need balance because you're not standing up.

So this is useful right?

Actually... no.

For starters, resistance machines of course have a place when it comes to teaching beginners to build muscle as well as helping people who are recovering from injury. If you have a damaged back then you might not be able to perform pull ups or squats with heavy weight. You can use mobility work to recover but in the *meantime* you should look for other ways to keep your other muscles strong. By completely isolating your muscles as you do in a resistance machine, you can completely remove any danger of hurting your back and thereby lift heavy weights.

But there's more. You see, if you're someone who is in excellent shape and who wants to perform like Bruce Lee, you can still injure yourself in the gym. In some ways, you're more likely too if you find yourself throwing about your one rep max.

Without a spotter, lifting a one rep max can actually be highly dangerous. I know a guy who fainted while pushing himself to the max on the bench press and if he hadn't have been with a spotter, then he'd have crushed himself.

Use Resistance Training To Build Strength You Can Actually Use

The whole point of a one rep max is that you can *barely move it*. This really isn't safe to lie underneath unless you have someone on hand to help!

And considering how important one rep maxes are for generating real strength, this creates an issue. You see where I'm going with this?

Because when you use a resistance machine, the weight is being held for you and thus it's completely safe. If you drop it, it has nowhere to fall and you can easily increase and decrease it even *during* your sets and reps.

This then also means you can perform overcoming isometrics with resistance machines. Just set it to a weight you can't move and *heave*.

This can be used in conjunction with your compound movements the end of a workout to strengthen your mind-muscle connection and to generally improve your raw strength.

Advanced Techniques With Resistance Machines

Performing overcoming isometrics isn't all you can do with resistance machines though. Another use for them is to vary your tempo.

You see, our muscles are actually stronger in one direction than the other. More specifically, they're stronger in the 'eccentric' phase of a movement, which is the portion where your muscle lengthens (versus the concentric, which is when the muscle shortens). This is when you lower the weight in most cases.

If you're stronger at lowering weights, then surely that means you should lift more during this portion of the movement right? Well yes, but it's not exactly easy with dumbbells!

On a resistance machine though, you can more easily get someone to help you lift a weight you can't move on your own (or even use the mechanism itself) and then lower it. On the chest press, you can even push out with both hands and then *lower* with just one hand effectively doubling the amount of weight you're moving. This is called 'eccentric overload' and it's an excellent way to really challenge your strength, while at the same time combining work for both the fast twitch and slow twitch muscle fiber.

Explode up, increase the weight and then lower through the count of five.

Chapter 9 – Movnat

A lesser-known but certainly no less cool fitness movement is that of 'MovNat'. MovNat means 'move natural' and it's all about doing exactly that: moving the way our bodies were designed to move in the environments that we were designed to move them in.

So what does this entail? It means climbing trees, it means trail running (barefoot of course), it means hopping across rocks and it means climbing cliff faces. It also means swimming in cold rivers (which by the way, has a ton of health benefits), throwing logs around and carrying other heavy objects long distances.

Not only is this kind of training a ton of fun but it's also very good for developing all kinds of motor skills that you probably don't even think about any more – like grip strength for climbing and forming calluses to toughen up.

Of course there are problems with too fully embracing this type of training too. One is that many of us aren't fortunate to have huge, sunny woodland to go running in. If you live somewhere cold and urban, then MovNat might mean running to the nearest park and splashing through mud in the rain.

Another issue here is of course the lack of instruction or structure. This is a pretty good way to get hurt and it's hard to know if you're progressing.

Don't completely embrace these movements then. Instead, just take from them what is useful. In the case of MovNat, remember that *anything* can be training and that there's a lot of good to be gained from just getting outside.

Start with structured training plans to restore your freedom of movement, your strength and your confidence. Once you've done this though, you should then start to experiment within your new movement framework. Don't be afraid to try new things and to *listen* to your body while you train. If something feels like a workout for the muscles, then it probably is. Who cares if you can't find it in a book anywhere?

Chapter 10 – Diet For Functional Strength

No training advice would be complete without a section on diet though. So to get the most functional fitness and power, you need to make sure you're eating right too.

What kind of diet advice goes well with functional training? Well, the most obvious 'fit' is yet another popular 'health fad'. This time we're looking at the Paleo diet. We're moving primal, so why not *eat* primal too?

What is the Paleo Diet?

The general concept behind the paleo diet is that you should eat as closely as possible to whatever you would eat in the wild. That means you shouldn't be eating anything that comes from a wrapper, or anything that has lots of additives in it.

It also actually means that you end up eating far fewer carbs. Think about it: how often would you come across a bowl of pasta in the wild? Or a loaf of bread? Our main source of carbohydrates in the wild were fruits and vegetables. Fruits might be rich in sugar but they're also a *fantastic* source of vitamins, minerals and other crucial nutrients that work wonders for the body. Vegetables meanwhile are slower to release their sugar but fuel us with just as many crucial nutrients.

The rest of the diet? Well that comes from meat of course! And this is great news for anyone looking to build functional strength as meat is where we get our amino acids – which are the building blocks of muscle.

Better yet, a truly paleo diet doesn't just eat any old meat but will seek out a lot of organ meat. In the wild, you wouldn't have been fussy about eating the heart or liver! Again, this is smart today as well because organ meat happens to be jam packed with all sorts of crucial nutrients.

If you follow this basic diet: eating more meat, more organ meat, more fruit and more vegetables – then you will feel healthier and more powerful than you ever have done.

Don't believe me? Then take a look at all the superfoods and supplements that everyone is raving about right now. You have CoEnzyme Q10 for example which increases mitochondrial function (you remember these guys from the chapter on HIIT?). So too does PQQ, l-carnitine, lutein and several other key ingredients.

Then you have things like omega 3 fatty acids which help the cells to communicate and improves your joints. You have your testosterone boosters, your nootropic herbs and your vasodilators…

You can take all these supplements and you'll see some benefits but you'll also spend a fortune. Alternatively though, if you just eat balanced diet including all the natural ingredients we've discussed, you'll *get* all those things in your diet. Liver is packed with CoQ10 and l-carnitine for instance, as is beef. It even includes creatine – the bodybuilding supplement used to increase energy and add muscle mass.

This is no coincidence either: we *evolved* eating these things and our body adapted accordingly. Our food isn't made for us: we're made for our food. If you're eating Mars bars all day then you're filling your body with damaging sugar and tons of calories and you're not getting any nutritional benefit from it!

A Word of Caution – Don't Go too Far!

But do be smart about this. Once again, it's important not to become *too* enamored with any one method of eating, including the Paleo diet.

For starters, you'll likely go mad if you never have an ice cream and in all likelihood strict rules like this will cause you to give up on your training. Likewise, it's key to remember that some modern foods are actually pretty good for us. A protein shake sure isn't paleo but it is convenient! The same goes for vitamin supplements – no, they aren't as easily absorbed by the body – but they're handy to have around when you don't have time to make a smoothie.

And there's no reason to completely eliminate bread from your diet. The idea that we can't digest bread is actually completely unfounded and untrue for anyone who doesn't have a legitimate gluten allergy.

Chapter 11 – Conclusion: Creating Your Own Program

So now you hopefully have a pretty good idea about functional strength, how it works and how it's different from other forms of training. Hopefully you'll be excited by the prospect to start increasing your real-world strength and power and to move more freely without pain. It's worth putting in the effort, as you'll find every aspect of life becomes easy. Even your brain will feel sharper and more youthful!

But how do you put all of this together into a training program you can actually use?

To start with, you have your seven primal movements, which we assigned some specific movements, like so:

- Squatting – Squats, deadlifts, kettlebell swings
- Lunging – Lunges, side squats
- Bending – Deadlifts, sit ups, leg raises
- Pushing – Bench press, overhead press, push up
- Pulling – Pull up, row
- Gait– Jogging, running, walking
- Twisting – Heavy bag, twisting sit ups, cable woodchop

Finish with some overcoming isometrics and grip work – whether that means bending a bar or using a power twister or resistance machines. Precede the workout with foam rolling and end it with stretching.

Use Resistance Training To Build Strength You Can Actually Use

These exercises alone will prove enough for most people to create a workout that challenges every part of the body and that triggers the maximum anabolic response. Choose one from each of the seven movements and train for high weight and relatively low repetitions on the compound lifts (i.e. three sets of 10).

This means you'll be training your whole body rather than doing a 'split' but remember that this is the most effective way to train. Not only does it mean that you're involving more muscle and thereby triggering a bigger anabolic response – it also means that you're using your time more efficiently. Ultimately, this means that if you ever miss a session, it won't be so hard to get back into your routine. It also avoids scenarios where you go for two weeks without training your biceps!

This also means you only need to train 3 times a week. More and you risk taxing your central nervous system and causing injury.

On a fourth day and optional fifth day though, you're going to use 20 minutes of HIIT training to burn fat and increase your mitochondrial function and density.

Combine this with a little bodyweight training when you can't make it to the gym and plenty of protein and nutrients.

The last ingredient is time. Keep it up and soon you'll feel fitter, stronger and healthier than you possibly ever imagined.

Welcome to the world of functional strength.

Other Senior Health and Fitness Books by This Author

If you would like to read more about Senior Health and Fitness, here is a list of the <u>titles, CreateSpace links and descriptions:</u>

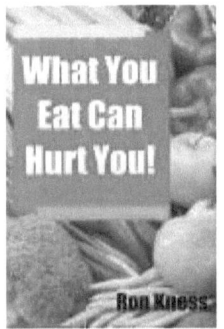

<u>What You Eat Can Hurt You</u>

https://www.createspace.com/4963196

Do you know that certain foods increase your risk for inflammation, disease and illness? It's true! And certain foods can help cure and heal you if you do get sick. Knowing which foods to eat and which ones to avoid empowers you to manage your own health.

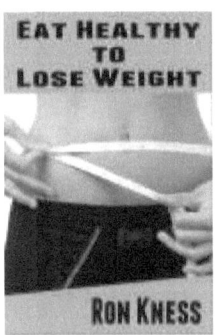

<u>Eat Healthy to Lose Weight</u>

https://www.createspace.com/4962939

As you read through our book, we show you which foods you should and should not be eating to reach your weight loss goal, along with discussing how to maintain your weight loss and stay within a few pounds of your goal weight. Banish the weight you keep gaining back each time by learning how to live a healthy lifestyle.

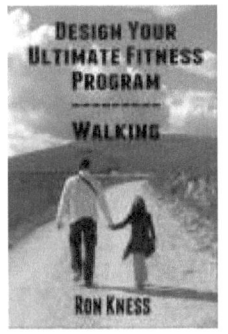

Design Your Ultimate Fitness Program - Walking

https://www.createspace.com/5252272

In my book Design Your Ultimate Fitness Program – Walking, we discuss the considerations that need to be made when designing a custom walking program, along with:

• Equipment needed
• Wearable technology you can use to track your walking
• And how to make walking more challenging

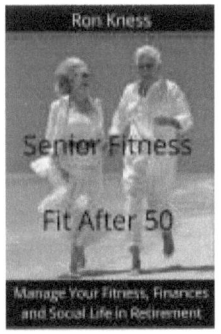

Senior Fitness – Fit After 50: Learn How to Manage Your Fitness, Finances and Social Life in Retirement

https://www.createspace.com/5474751

Inside you will discover answers to your most pressing questions:
• What do I need to know about downsizing my home?
• What are the best tips for staying healthy as you approach your 50's?
• When should I start planning for retirement?
• I am worried about being lonely once I retire, do others feel the same?

• Is it worthwhile to carry two homes during retirement?
And more…

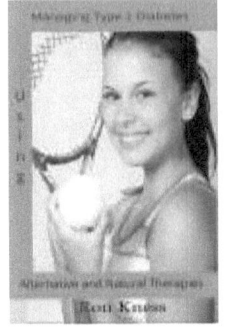

Managing Type 2 Diabetes Using Alternative And Natural Therapies

https://www.createspace.com/5401244

While Type 2 diabetes can be managed medically, there are many alternative natural and holistic methods of therapy and treatment that can further enhance quality of life and minimize the effects of this disease. In this book, I discuss 12 different types, including yoga, reflexology and acupuncture to name just three.

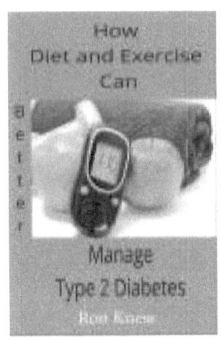

How Diet and Exercise Can Better Manage Type 2 Diabetes

https://www.createspace.com/5404845

Of the different types of diabetes, only Type 2 can be reversed. In my book How Diet and Exercise Can Better Manage Type 2 Diabetes, we reveal the three things you can do to best manage your disease, including:
• Diet
• Exercise
• Weight management

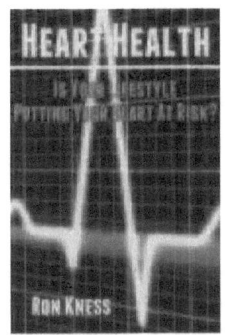

Heart Health: Is Your Lifestyle Putting Your Heart at Risk?

https://www.createspace.com/5464020

In my ebook Is Your Lifestyle Putting Your Heart At Risk? we discuss the six greatest risks to your heart and the lifestyle changes you can make to mitigate them.

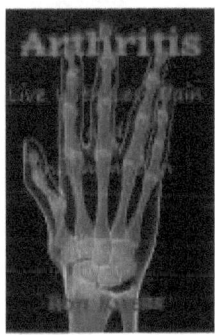

Arthritis – Live Wth Less Pain and Inflammation: Tips and Techniques You Can Use to Lessen the Pain and Inflammation

https://www.createspace.com/5457441

Discover Simple Tips & Information That Will Help Reduce The Painful Symptoms Of Arthritis!

You learn things like:
• Simple and effective information that will help you manage the pain and inflammation that comes along with arthritis, so that you can live an active, full life without debilitating pain.
• The different types of arthritis, their symptoms and how to alleviate their painful side effects.
• The pros and cons of over-the-counter arthritis medications, plus simple tips that will help you know how to choose the right supplements.
• Free, yet effective ways to get relief from arthritis pain and

inflammation, so you don't have to suffer anymore.
the effects arthritis can have significant impact on your physical and mental well-being, but this books shows you how to overcome its painful symptoms and live life relatively pain free.

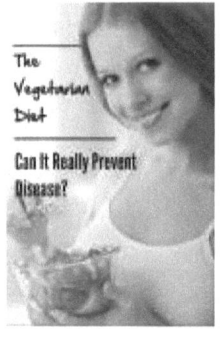

The Vegetarian Diet – Can It Really Prevent Disease?

https://www.createspace.com/5519874

Is a vegetarian diet right for you? Multiple studies have shown over and over that a vegetarian diet goes along way in preventing certain chronic diseases, such as:

• Heart Disease
• Cancer
• Diverticulitis
• Type 2 Diabetes
• Hypertension
• Obesity
• Kidney Failure

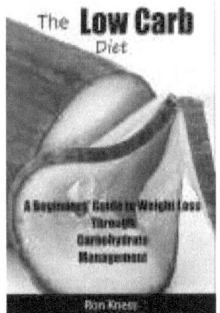

The Low Carb Diet: A Beginner's Guide to Weight Loss Through Carbohydrate Management

https://www.createspace.com/5416348

In my book "The Low-Carb Diet – A Beginners' Guide to Weight Loss Through Carbohydrate Management", I reveal a successful method of losing weight based in part on the amount and type of carbohydrates you consume.

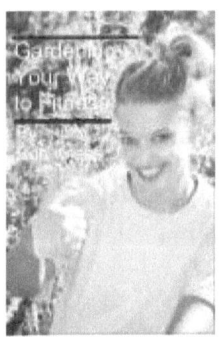

Gardening Your Way to Fitness: The Fun Way to Get Fit and Provide Beauty and Healthful Bounty for Your Family

https://www.createspace.com/5459564

The gym is a great place to stay fit during the colder seasons, but once the temperature turns warmer you want to spend more time outside. Plus, you'll have the benefit of fresh wholesome produce to enjoy by growing vegetables in your backyard garden.

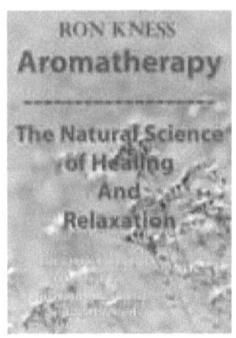

Aromatherapy - The Science of Healing and Relaxation: Learn How Essential Oils Elicit The Relaxation Response And Alter Mood

https://www.createspace.com/5714434

In my book Aromatherapy – The Science of Healing and Relaxation, we reveal the natural holistics methods you can use to heal the body from certain medical issues and to relive stress through relaxation. In particular we talk about:

• Aromatherapy - what it is and how it works
• Essential Oils – how the effects of certain aromas differs from others
• Recipes – how to make your own essential oil combinations

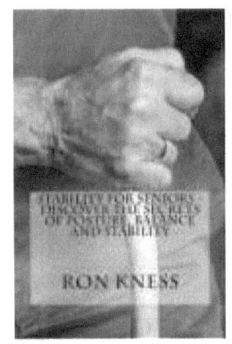

Stability for Seniors: Discover the Secrets of Posture, Balance and Stability

https://www.createspace.com/6096479

Many people sacrifice their health in pursuit of their career. They are so busy making a living that they neglect to make a life. The excuse that they do not have time to exercise is tossed about so frequently that they end up letting their health and fitness slide.

If you are not regularly active, you will have muscular atrophy over time. Your flexibility will decrease. Your core strength will diminish. As time progresses, you will be less limber and more rigid.

Use Resistance Training To Build Strength You Can Actually Use

This is exactly how people age poorly. It's a process that has snowballed over time.

Only with regular exercise and a healthy diet can you have a body that is fit and has the ability to almost reverse aging.

If you have neglected your health for years and life seems to be a chore now because you can't get around without assistance, do not feel dejected.

You can remedy the situation. You can restore the strength, balance and stamina that you have lost. It is never too late to become what you might have been.

This guide will show you exactly what you need to do to restore your balance, strengthen your core and give you the ability to live life to its fullest. Read how ...

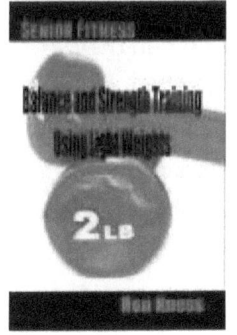
Senior Fitness – Balance and Strength Training Using Light Weights

https://www.createspace.com/6107842

As you age you notice that you are not as strong as before. Most of us simply chalk that up to the "natural" aging process. However, to fight the physical dangers of aging, strength is very important.

The problem is that each and every debilitating and even deadly issues can be positively impacted by simply lifting light weights, yet seniors are not strength training.

The following are the incredible benefits of simply lifting light weights a few times each week for seniors ...

* A feeling of self-esteem and self-confidence

* Improved circulatory system

* Lowered risk of heart disease

* Regulation of a naturally healthy body weight

* Light weightlifting is an effective way to treat and eradicate back pain

* You have fewer feelings of depression, anxiety and stress

* You strengthen your bones, naturally improving your ability to fight health issues like osteoporosis

* Light weightlifting is excellent for preventing and treating diabetes

* Arthritis sufferers experience fewer painful symptoms when they weight train regularly

* Your balance and flexibility are boosted, and joint pain is reduced.

By now you are probably sold on the fact that you need to be lifting light weights and strength training if you are over 50 years of age or older.

So, what's your next step?

Reserve your copy of this book that shows you exactly how to benefit from lifting light weights as a senior citizen.

About the Author

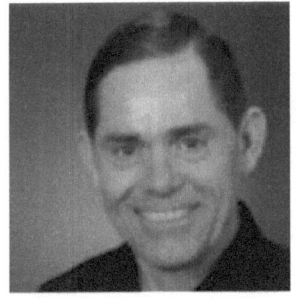

I grew up in Central Minnesota, where my parents own and operated a fishing resort. Once out of high school I tried a couple of semesters of college, only to quit halfway through the Spring term; I decided at that time that college wasn't for me.

Then I decided to follow my father's previous occupation as an auto mechanic. I graduated from a two-year of vocational training course and worked as a mechanic. While in vocational training, I decided to join the National Guard where I eventually ended up working full-time for 32 years.

So how does all of this relate to writing? In one of my leadership schools, the instructor, who was an English teacher at a juvenile detention center, presented writing to me in a whole new way - a way that started to develop my interest in working with words.

Fast forward about 40 years and I now have over 50 books listed on Amazon for Kindle and CreateSpace.